Over the Rainbow.....
finding Happiness with bipolar

By

Cathie Temple

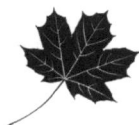

MAPLE
PUBLISHERS

Over the Rainbow..... finding Happiness with bipolar

Author: Cathie Temple

Copyright © 2025 Cathie Temple

The right of Cathie Temple to be identified as author of this work has been asserted by the author in accordance with section 77 and 78 of the Copyright, Designs and Patents Act 1988.

First Published in 2025

ISBN 978-1-83538-602-6 (Paperback)
      978-1-83538-683-5 (E-Book)

Book Cover Design and Book Layout by:
      White Magic Studios
      www.whitemagicstudios.co.UK

Published by:
      Maple Publishers
      Fairbourne Drive, Atterbury,
      Milton Keynes,
      MK10 9RG, UK
      www.maplepublishers.com

A CIP catalogue record for this title is available from the British Library.

All rights reserved. No part of this book may be reproduced or translated in any form or by any means, electronic or mechanical, including photocopying, recording or by any information storage and retrieval system without written permission from the author.

The views expressed in this work are solely those of the author and do not necessarily reflect the publisher's opinions, and the publisher, as a result of this, disclaims any responsibility for them.

CONTENTS

Cathie

This is my story. Growing up with bipolar.

37 house moves and 4 &1/2 husbands!

Rising to my best self,
and finding happiness.

Foreword

Google states bipolar disorder is a mental health condition that causes extreme mood swings, from hypermania to severe depression. After an episode of mania, the depression could become devastating, leading to the loss of trust and love in close relationships.

Medicines and counselling can help.

I had no idea bipolar was in my family.

Apparently, it is usually diagnosed in people in their twenties.

I was 29 and had been divorced for 4 years.

And I was living in Australia.

In my personal experience I became very excited and headstrong. I felt psychic and elated but soon experienced madness, thinking and doing things that could have been fatal to me.

I think this explains why I was constantly seeking a true friend and partner to support me, as friends didn't always understand.

This is my journey...

Trusting and loving myself

Riding the downs and dancing in the highs

And finding True Love.

Chapter 1

My childhood

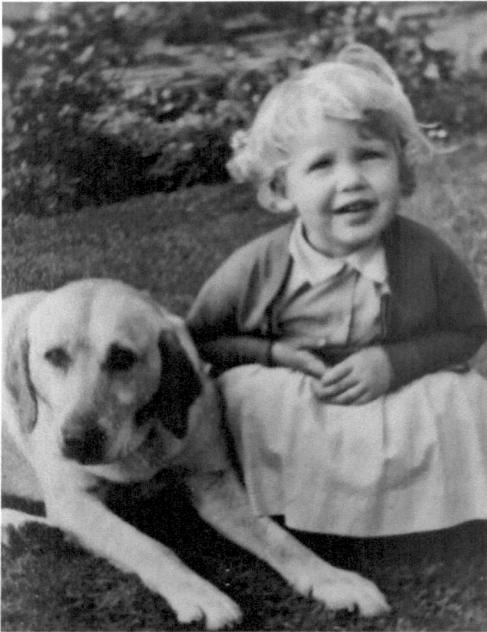

Cathie

I was born Anne Catherine Turnbull, 18th February 1958 in Woking, Surrey. The first baby born to Adam and Jo. I was very loved, even though my Dad found it hard to understand me.

My Dad was born in 1923, a very different world to the 60s, of Rock and Roll and the Beatles. Mum had several miscarriages before I came along. Some would say I was reluctant to come into this world.

Mum said I was a difficult child. But I think I just wanted to dance and express myself, as I did when I visited my grandmother on their farm near Bournemouth. It was heaven down there for me. Grampa had Friesian cows, two lovely dogs and kittens in the barn.

Our family lived in Loughton, Essex, a London suburb on the central line. It was a nice, detached house, but very 70s, rather dull and uninviting. We did have a gorgeous garden though, with a huge willow tree and a large vegetable patch for my Dad to tender.

My father was a kind and loving man, but being a senior consultant at the London Hospital, Whitechapel, he would come home very tired and could not bear upset easily. Consequently, the family had to be silent when he returned from work until after he had started his dinner.

At various times after some such upset I would be sent to my bedroom with a closed door and told not to come down. I would wait in in floods of tears until he would be ready to ask me downstairs, but never any discussion, sympathy or explanation, which left me always trying to impress in other ways.

He relaxed at weekends, in the garden or out sailing. As a young teenager I could think of nothing worse than going out on the boat and only accompanied the family when I had to. If it was hot, I would spend the entire trip sunbathing while my mother diligently took command of the rudder!

I loved my Barbies when I was young. Later I enjoyed cycling everywhere, drawing and making models.

My parents gave me a small portable record player and bought me all the new Beatles singles - wish I'd kept them!

I loved animals. We had a basset hound called Becky who was a great character and had energy fits, racing round the garden about once a month.

When I was about seven, after some upset with my parents, I put Becky on her lead and walked towards Epping Forest. It must've been very worrying for my parents, but my Dad found me and brought me home. I remember him giving me a stern talk in our downstairs loo. It was very dangerous at that time as there had been a couple of murders in the forest.

My brother was born Stuart Richard on May 19, 1962. Blonde, blue eyed and full of energy! Overall, we got on well, though I do remember us having a bad fight one day when Stuart pulled some of my hair out! Stuart is musical and very sporty. Completely opposite to me. Though I love my music I don't play an instrument. I did learn to play the piano at prep school, but it didn't come naturally.

When I was six, I remember altering a quiz at kindergarten to say that I had won a competition. When my mother picked me up, I ran to her shouting "Mummy, mummy, look I have won!" only to be discovered that I had lied, and a visit from the headmistress to my mother's sitting room resulted in tears.

I liked being at home with Mum. She was a lovely person, warm and approachable. I was creative but often bored. I did love entering a competition or two, and winning sometimes, even the BBC 'Go to work on an Egg'. I also had a Blue Peter badge.

Mum was a great cook and always provided us with good wholesome meals. She had been a nurse before she met Dad, then part-time for a local hospital, and was on a couple of charity committees. She baked Dad a cake every week.

When I was about 13 my Dad had an extension built over our garage. This was my teenage bedroom. It was quite big and had a little bar where I put a kettle. I asked if I could paint the long wall down the far side. I chose a bright blue and orange, and painted large flowers, ...so 70's. I had a blue carpet to match. I felt very modern, especially wearing my trendy Hot pants and white platform shoes, which I had begged my Mum to buy for me!

When Jesus Christ Superstar the pop opera was released, I copied all the lyrics and sang along to it constantly. I love it to this day.

My grandmother moved near us in Loughton after my grandfather died. It was hard for her. They had had a marvellous life running a hotel in Bournemouth and then running a dairy farm in Bexhill on Sea. I was very close to her. She was a beautiful soul. Even in her last years she baked cakes for Mum and made sweets shaped like fruits for local charities.

She died when she was 88, sitting in her favourite chair at Christmas time, dressed up and holding a glass of sherry. What a way to go!

I remember her dearly at the farm in Bexhill, me holding a little mushroom basket and her singing 'Happiness', Ken Dodd's signature song. I must've been about 2!

Mum and Dad took my brother and I on holiday every summer, first Cornwall ... then France a few times, then onto Spain and Italy. It was in Italy my life really changed.... but that was after Riddlesworth ....

—◦━◖◗━◦—

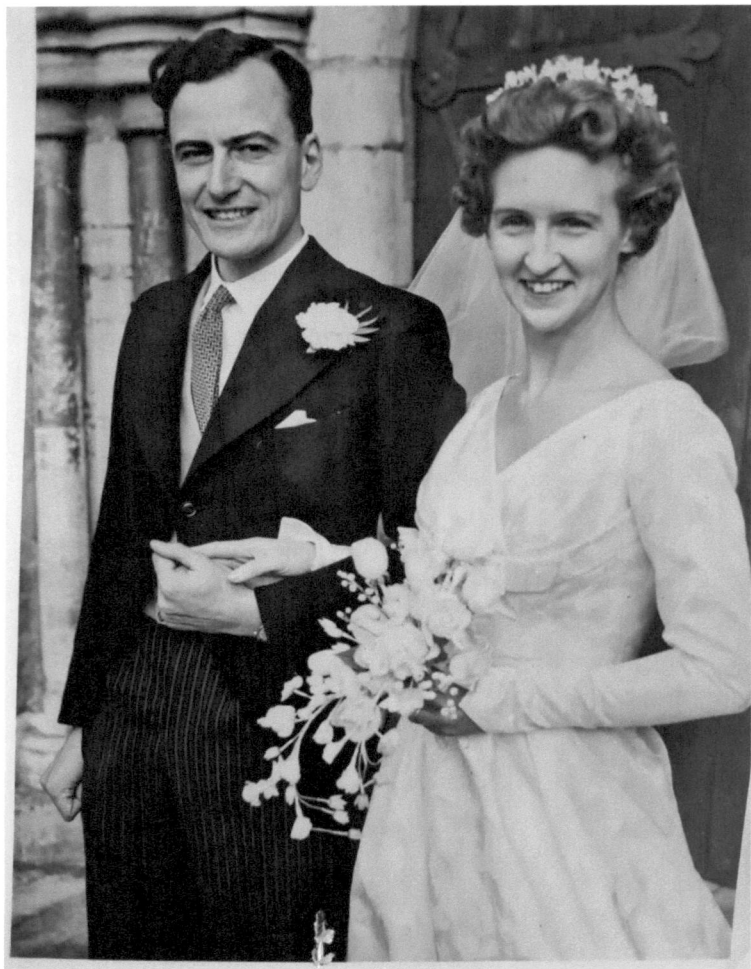

Mum and Dad 1956

Chapter 2

School

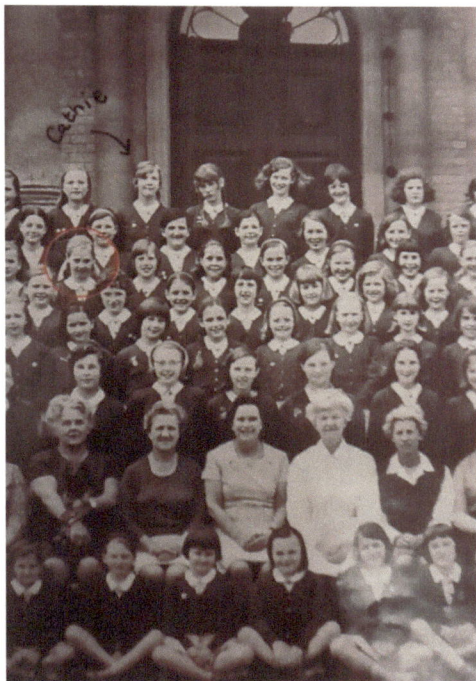

Riddlesworth Hall 1971
(Diana circled in red)

When I was eight, I was sent to Riddlesworth Hall, an all- girls boarding school in Norfolk. This was a complete shock and resulted in many tears, trying to get used to the change.

When I started at Riddlesworth, I was nicknamed "sorry". This makes me feel sad for the little girl I was, taken away from her home and her parents, aged 8.

This is the same prep school that Princess Diana attended although she was three years younger than me. I only remember her as a new pupil when I was made Head girl at age 12.

My parents had put me down for this school soon after I was born. They had both been boarders and loved it.

As Head girl I was expected to monitor the dormitories at night with my prefects and hold meetings for the whole school every week. We sat on highchairs with the whole school sitting in front of us on the floor. I was in the middle and had to report on pupils' behaviour and forthcoming events. I'm sure this wouldn't happen now.

The headmistress, Miss Ridsdale, was the Art teacher. She was fair and extremely likeable.

I had my paintings all over the Art room walls. Suddenly the talent of my grandfather had come through with all the help and encouragement of this lovely lady. I wasn't especially liked by the other teachers; I was cheeky and naughty, but I had developed an independence, and I got on well with the other girls. Unfortunately I suffered from lack of confidence and an eating disorder started to emerge which lasted on and off until I was about 35. At this stage I put stones in my pockets when being weighed, later bulimia took over ...I think a result of wanting to be accepted and low self-esteem.

I loved fashion and made many drawings of models, clothes and hairstyles ... I dreamt of going to Art college after school, but Miss Ridsdale (Riddy) advised my parents of drugs and debauchery there, so unfortunately that never happened!

Over time I did get close to an attractive, sporty girl called Debbie .... we spent all our free time together, wrote notes and love letters, but when I had to go to hospital to have my tonsils out, she wanted nothing to do with me. She had another best friend, it was devastating. I had never known the pain of loving and losing ... a state I would have to go through many times in my life.

I was only about 11or 12.

I was 13 when I started at a new boarding school, Queenwood in Hertfordshire. There were no good Art facilities here, and I became very restless and bored. I did have two lovely friends though, and we started smoking and skipping lessons. One day we made a Ouija board.

I had been reading books like Daughters of Satan by Jean Plaidy, and I was curious of the occult. One of my friends had lost her father previously. We apparently connected with him. The glass moved to answer all her questions, she was obviously upset and ran off....It was a surreal experience and opened my mind to other realms. But this experience was not something I wanted to repeat, I felt scared and very confused.

One day, while roaming the grounds, I met a boy called Frank. His school, Haileybury, adjoined ours, and he had crossed over for a walk. Frank's family lived in Reading, and I was in invited to my first outdoor Pop festival when I was 14. it was so fantastic, Sun, music, teenagers hanging out on the street. I didn't want the day to end. We tried to see each other when we could, and even went to the Dorchester Hotel in London for a Ball. I remember the lime green halter neck dress I wore on that summer evening. It felt magical.

We didn't see each other for long, but a few years later he turned up at my Mum 's house in Loughton and asked after me... much to his surprise Mum told him I was married!

My parents realised how unhappy I was, and I resumed my O- Levels at a high school in Loughton. It was a completely different experience! An all-girls school, boyfriends, and motorbikes, not the upmarket schools I had been used to. I went to see Status Quo at Finsbury Park, greyhound racing, and my first (and last) football match.

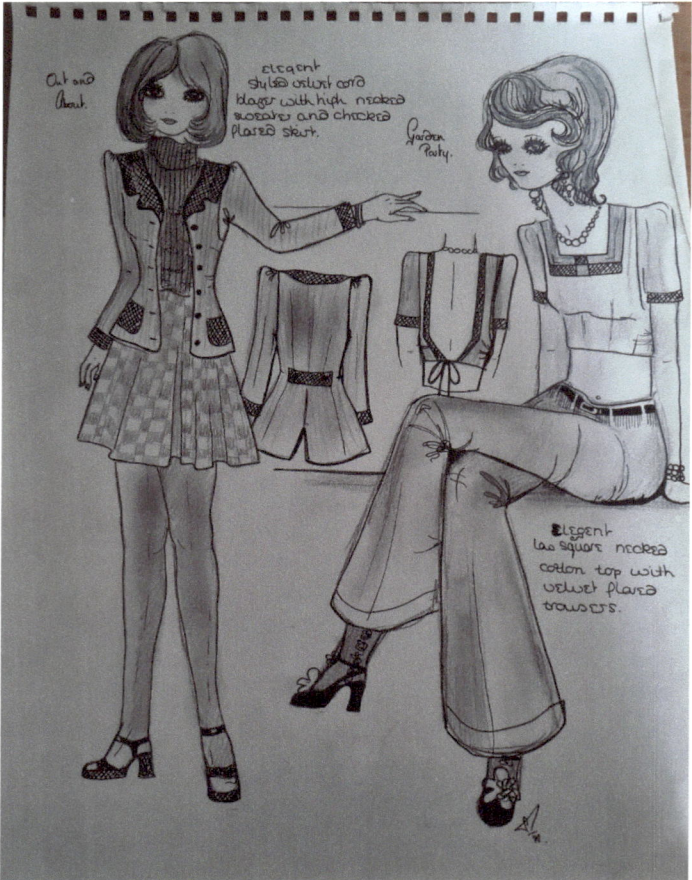

Original drawing age 14

Chapter 3

London

When I left school, I couldn't wait to live in London, my mother helped me find a flat. I was 16. I was to live with medical students who she thought would be a good influence. Unfortunately, they soon saw through the age difference. They were 18! I had to move.

I wasn't happy in the cookery class or the secretarial course my mother had booked for me. Or the girl's dormitory. I ended up on the till in the Great American Disaster, a trendy hamburger restaurant nearby in Beauchamp Place, round the corner from Harrods. I worked with a group of wonderful gay waiters who danced down the aisle singing to disco tracks! One evening I got taken to see Barry White at the Royal Albert Hall by a young customer and his parents. It was great, we had a Box and looked down on the stage. Barry and his orchestra were fabulous, and we laughed to see many ladies in the stalls throwing their underwear at him!

Soon after I applied for a job in Monsoon, a stylish boutique nearly opposite the restaurant. A young chap who assisted the managers had to come to the window of the Disaster to check whether I looked okay to be working in the in the boutique! I began working in Monsoon with Emma Jacobs, daughter of David, the radio personality, and was suddenly in my element. In those days we often sat on bean bags on the floor. We were allowed to smoke and wear the lovely Indian clothes and jewellery from the shop. It was so relaxed and very bohemian. Things did change after a few years and the shop had to become more formal.

At this point it was quite an exclusive store with celebrities like Jane Seymour modelling for us in Kashmir for our advertisements.

At first, I was worried I'd never be able to talk to customers with the ease of my manager Emma, but soon my confidence grew.

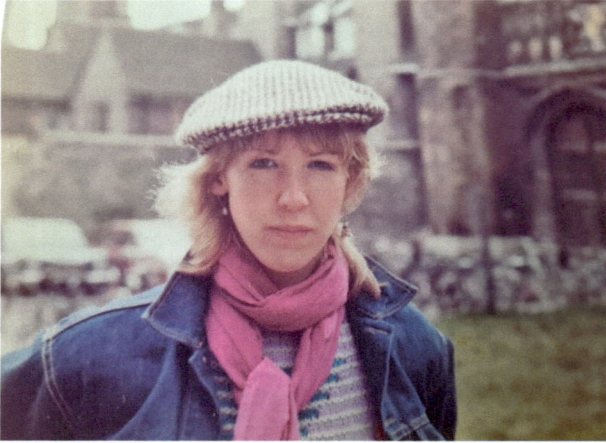

Cathie age 20

Chapter 4

Jonathan

A couple of years earlier I had met a boy on holiday in Italy, when camping with my parents. His name was Jonathan.

I fell in love almost immediately. I had been longing to have a proper boyfriend for years, even though I was only fifteen.

Any time I got the opportunity I would try and make it happen and this time was no exception. I was on the lookout.

One evening I came across a table of young people with their parents having their dinner outside, so I stopped to say hello. There were two very nice-looking boys in the party, so I sat down near them. Very soon after this meeting I got together with one of the boys. It was really like love at first sight. It was 1973, the days of Led Zeppelin and Stairway to Heaven. We kissed on the beach; we didn't care about anybody. The parents of the other boy who had taken them all on holiday were very doubtful that anything would last. On The last day of the holiday Jo drove me to Florence in his beat-up Fiat 500. What a thrill!

On return we kept in contact; we lived on opposite sides of London but that didn't deter us. We had no mobile phones so it was only done through the telephone and making sure we got to see each other as often as we could. Jo was at college, and I was planning to live in London, so we managed to work things out.

Unfortunately, the last few years of school had left me with anorexia and bulimia - an eating disorder. I had heard from somebody that it was possible to lose weight by making yourself sick after meals. The inability to really open myself up to my parents had left scars, coupled with insecurities from boarding school.

Regardless of this, I was happy to be in London and confident on my path. I did break up from Jo for a short while but when I realised how difficult it was to meet anybody and get on my feet in London, we soon got back together again. We lived together for a year before we decided to get married and buy a house. I was 18.

Working at Monsoon was good. I became a manager and eventually opened the new store in London's Covent Garden.

We went to see musicals and the latest films. One evening in 1973, we went to see a new show at the Royal Court Theatre, Sloane Sq. The Rocky Horror Show was truly a revelation and an eye opener for whoever attended. We had never seen partial nudity on stage or men dressed as women in such an outrageous fashion!

I remember travelling to work on the tube and seeing many funky, bohemian people and not knowing how to meet them. We did go to gigs, but our main friends weren't very open minded. We saw films, went to bars and had dinner parties. It took a few years to meet a different type of crowd.

Unfortunately, being married did not cure my bulimia. I hid it as best I could from work and from Jo and friends. I hated myself for letting it happen, but it didn't happen every day and I had a routine that I knew how to handle.

By this time, I was enjoying working in Covent Garden. It was very exciting as the market had just been reopened and there were some wonderful shops and events going on. I had lovely staff, and I enjoyed this position tremendously. Jo and I went out with friends in London quite a bit but I couldn't confide in him.. I didn't really know who I was at that stage or what I really wanted in the long run. Jo had always dreamt of having a garage of his own and children, but I didn't feel ready. It wasn't that I didn't want children; it was just not in my vision for that time.

I wanted to travel and meet people. We did travel to the Greek islands and drove through America on the Greyhound bus on one holiday, which we loved.

Unfortunately, we were quite different and as the years went by, I got more and more frustrated, and the tell-tale signs of unhappiness began to show. One evening, out with friends, Jo told me that he couldn't live with me anymore. It was a total shock. At the time there was no changing the situation, he had made up his mind. Later he did ask whether we could make it work, but too much had happened by then and I realised we wanted very different paths.

I remember sitting up on the couch in our living room, looking out of the window, crying my heart out. As I stared through the window, I wondered if I would ever be happy again.

I had to create a life on my own.

⋯⊷⊰◈⊱⊶⋯

Chapter 5

Australia

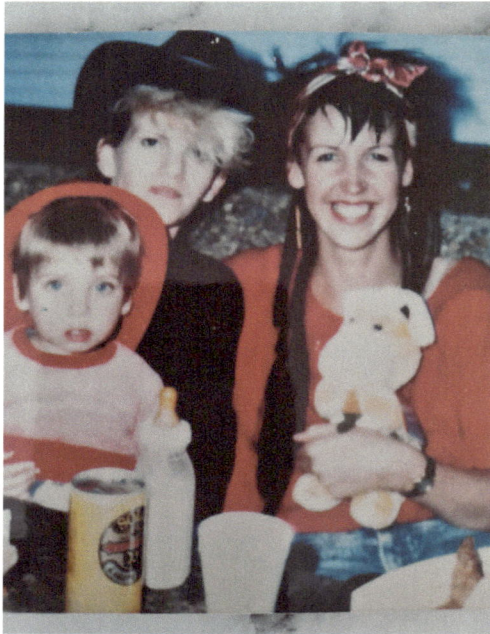

Sydney 1983

I was 24 and alone …. Fear gripped me. I couldn't even go to work without bursting into tears. Eventually my manager, who was very worried about me, suggested that I might like to go to Perth, Australia to help open a new Monsoon branch. I was going with the flow, a dream come true, but I hadn't dreamt of anything like this. I was a bit scared but optimistic too. My parents were very supportive, and I made it to the to the flight, stopping at Bali for a week on the way.

I'd never taken drugs before but in Bali I was offered a magic mushroom omelette and that was the beginning of my dalliance with a few substances..... I couldn't stop writing as I sat under a beautiful palm tree in this fantastically tropical country, and in the balmy evening dusk I just wrote and wrote. I obviously needed to cleanse myself of everything that had happened over the last six or so years.

When I arrived in Perth, I got picked up by a lady who had been my manager in Monsoon for a year or two previously. Dianne was 12 years older than I and from Australia herself. I suddenly went from being the manageress of the Covent Garden branch, which I had worked up to all that time, to being a humble shop girl again. It was strange and I didn't know anybody, but I was just absorbing the beauty of the country. The wonderful plants and flowers, the beach, the sky and the people.

I developed a horrible eczema rash on my hands and face. I was shedding a skin, I guess, but my manageress was not impressed. I moved out and found a small flat near the shop. I felt free.

There was a boy who was working outside the shop. I think he was a builder and he asked me out. I was so nervous I said no, but after a few days I realised that it would be lovely to connect with somebody.

He was sweet and calm and tanned. I began a relationship with him, meeting all his friends and he helped me move into a little flat. It all went very well. I had three months helping open this branch and when I had to go home it was quite sad to leave him and his friends.

When I got home, I knew I just wanted to be back in Australia. Friends had told me that Sydney was amazing, so I took a flight there. I had a connection in the city of a friend I'd met in Perth, so I knew where to start.

Sydney Wow! Sydney in the 80's. What a city. I ended up in King's Cross where the street girls hung out on the pavements and there were loads of bars and clubs. Behind the main drag, Darlinghurst Road, there were lovely trees and flowering plants. I just loved the buzz, and it was a cheap area.

I found a flat share down here on Bayswater Road. My room was huge, and I had two very colourful flatmates. One trendy boy called Richard, who was in love with an older girl called Robin, who lived in the adjoining flat, and another boy. I think they liked me because I was from London and felt I was cool in that way. They kind of looked after me.

After a while I met a girl called Angie. She had had some bad things happen to her, like me, and we hit it off. She worked as a cocktail waitress at a club down the road. I felt happy again.

I found a job in a café in Kellett St, very close, but soon got bored and took a new job helping sell crafts and paintings in a trendy gallery on the same street. Such fun.

We had David Bowie 's China girl living across the road. We used to see her and her friends having parties on the patio, everyone wearing white, listening to Sade. One day she came into the gallery.

She was softly spoken and very beautiful. It was a great thrill, but we didn't dare ask her about David! We listened to Boy George, Duran Duran and disco... we danced at clubs whenever we could. The 80's!

I met a wonderful girl called Silvia in the gallery. She made beautiful clothes, and we sold some of them for her. She and I went out quite a bit and it was so lovely to have a sincere friendship. Silvia is from Italy and now Sydney is her home. She has become a lifelong friend who I am still in contact with today.

One evening I returned home from working at the café and realised I'd forgotten my keys. It must've been about midnight.... I called my flatmate, but I had to wait till he got back from work. King's Cross was not a place you'd want to hang out on your own, but I was naïve. I waited on the wall opposite my flat on Bayswater Rd. It was dark except for a couple of streetlamps.

This strange, tramp like man walked up to me and started talking. I didn't think anything of it until he produced a broken bottle from his pocket. It was horrifying. He took my arm and began to lead me towards a dark alley. I knew I might get hurt if he continued.

I gabbled. I talked about my Mum and Dad and told him they'd miss me. I prayed to God. I was completely in fear of my life. Then suddenly two people appeared from the shadows .... I just shook him off and ran! I screamed all the way to my building and thankfully someone let me in.

I was incredibly lucky.

I remember moving to a small flat in in a new area. I joined a drama class, but it wasn't for me. I couldn't act at all, but I met some nice people.; I hardly knew who I was.

One evening, I went to a play and met an animated boy who said he was an actor. I eventually got to know him better, but it didn't work out as a relationship. I couldn't help acting like I was married and wanted to see him all the time. That wasn't cool, so in the end he broke my heart, and I started drawing cards and using his name, which I changed from Kerry to Perry, and I made my Perry cards. I ended up having these printed and selling in Sydney and Melbourne. It was a conscious revenge really. I did wonder how it affected him, until I heard he had gone to prison in New Zealand for cannabis misuse.

I had a stall at Paddington market, a riot of colour and young designers making their own clothes and furniture. It was a wonderful time. A friend made me some poles so I could display my T-shirts which I had had printed. It was just so great to have a purpose, to have a way of expressing my art. My character Perry was like a 20-year-old guy in dark shades and a sweater, the image I got from Charlie Brown. My Dad was very fond of the Peanuts cartoon books which I'd seen growing up.

Kerry was very profound. One quote I got from him was "it's so hard being a bi-sexual actor in Sydney"! So, Perry was to be a would-be actor too. Trendy and a deep thinker, he liked sitting in coffee shops contemplating the World!

Later, my animation also included a cat called Psyche.

I took my designs to Melbourne and sold some cards into a few cafes. Everybody was so friendly, and I really enjoyed the city.

While I was at the market, I was approached by a TV company interested in making a film about me and my character Perry. It was such fun. My grannie had made a cotton jumper just like Perry wore, and one of our friends, who was an actor, copied his outfit and played his part. In the film I was arranging my t-shirts when my friend came up and surprised me as Perry. It was very funny, and was first shown on a children's show, similar to Blue Peter.

After a year or so and lots of work designing and selling at the market I did show my work to a card company. Problem being it was just a bit too sarcastic. I was trying to be funny, but it didn't quite pay off. But what did happen was that a friend went to Auckland and saw my T-shirt designs in a department store over there. Unfortunately, I hadn't been able to patent my work in New Zealand - only in Australia, so there was nothing I could do.

But I must say it was a good indication that my work had had an impression on people, and somebody was bothered enough to have my designs copied and taken to the shops over there.

I felt good about that.

I have always been interested in psychics and tarot. One day in Sydney I went to see two readers I had heard were good.

When they were reading for me, their faces darkened. They said very difficult times were ahead, but I would blossom in my later years. Recently I have wondered if the dark days they mentioned were about Covid. They also told me I would write a book, and since then I have been waiting for the right time. Now, all this time later, I feel I have something worth writing about.

Life wasn't always plain sailing. I did get very moody and at one stage got quite depressed. I was always trying to find another boyfriend but none of my associations seem to last long. I dabbled in a few drugs; the worst time was when I met a guy who asked me whether I'd like to try heroin. I can't imagine now why I would to have wanted to do that, but I had little resistance. I had smoked some at a party and found it extremely pleasant. One night he injected me. I was violently sick and swore never to let that happen again. I was quite depressed at this time... I think friendships had changed and I felt very lonely and lost.

During this time, I did go up and down quite a lot. Changing flats, changing boyfriends. I did take

LSD a couple of times and enjoyed it. I saw the world differently and a spiritual side of me that I connected with helped me understand the bad times. I read a book called Out on a Limb by Shirley MacLaine and everything seemed to make sense. Things happen for a reason and looking at the signs I was beginning to sort out who I was and what I could achieve. Sometimes I felt very powerful, especially having new ideas and creating my work.

Sometimes I would go the other way but was able to pull myself back.

I would fly around on my bike all over Sydney. I had taken driving tests in England but never got my licence. Jo would drive us in London. I always became very anxious about the test and subsequently failed every time. It was fun cycling with the wind in my hair!

One adventure I had was when a couple of friends asked me to join them driving up the coast to Uluru (Ayres Rock) and climbing it. Nowadays the Aboriginals don't let visitors do that, as it is their sacred land. We had a gruelling time getting to the top. I remember my friend Roger, who managed the Valhalla cinema in Sydney, cheering madly when we got there. It was so windy, but we had an incredible view over the desert.

We drove up the coast up to the Northern Territory ... one time the car broke down and I had to go into a hotel (pub), full of men to ask for help.

There was one lady behind the bar, just like in Priscilla, Queen of the Desert, and she was scary. But we were successful and someone helped us. We made it to Alice Springs and Darwin. I had fake black dreads at the time and did look very strange to the locals. I met one lovely young Aboriginal man who told me about their struggles but also how much he loved his culture. It was sad to see so many finding it difficult to cope.

Back in Sydney, it was still hot. I joined some friends about 5am and headed to the beach. They were smoking some strong Marijuana and as I walked to the sea, I felt I was walking on the water; I think I was tripping. After this I went off on my own, spotting a small tree I took my clothes off, curled up and dreamt I was in the garden of Gethsemane, no one saw me. I did some other very strange things. I walked with two gay guys along the road and invited myself into their house. Later I strolled into a police station and thought I was on candid camera! Eventually the police saw what was going on and helped me back to my flat.

My flatmate was very concerned about me because she could see I wasn't well and took me to the hospital. I was in a state of psychosis. In the hospital they gave me an injection and I slept and slept. I was probably there at least a week or two, but I wasn't given any medication. I can't remember feeling scared or unhappy. Just glad of the rest, I think.

One day I was allowed to see The Never-Ending Story at the cinema. I was blown away by the story; in my state it all meant something significant and meaningful.

When I got back to my flat, I arranged to go home to London. I remember thinking that I'd been over in Sydney a long time and I needed to reconnect with my parents. I didn't mind leaving my friends and going home, but I didn't know how difficult it would be when I got back to England.

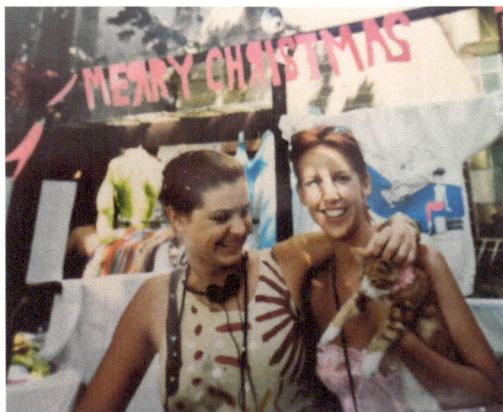

Paddington Market 1985

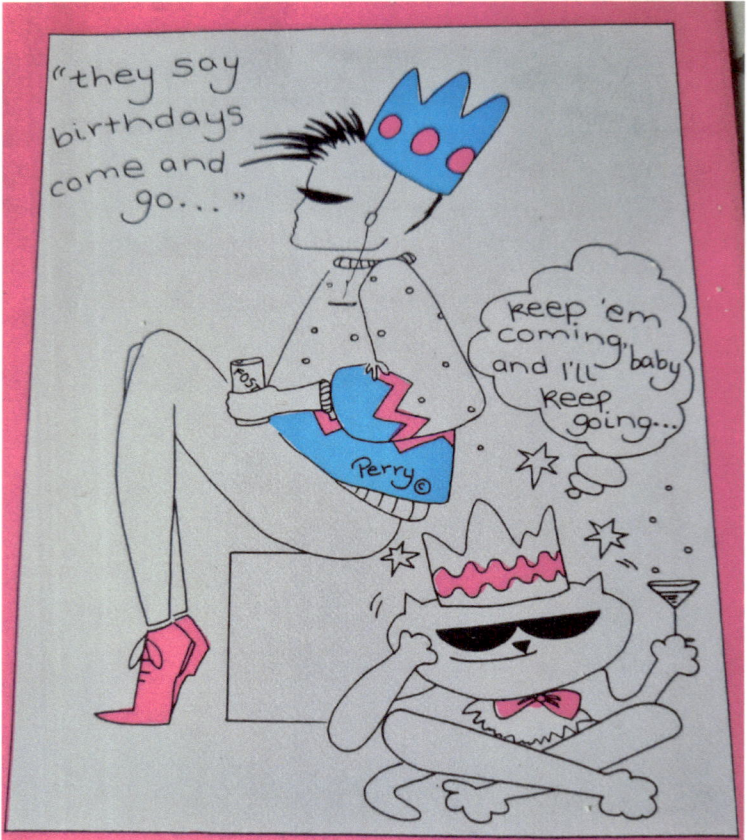

'Perry' card

Chapter 6

Returning Home

I felt better. I managed to pack up what I could and fly home. It was nice to see my parents but I very soon realized I would have to get out and find work. At that time Loughton was very uninspiring. I felt much better in myself and couldn't wait to be in London again.

I got a job at Anokhi as a manageress and my Dad helped me kit out a little flat in Ladbroke Grove.

At first all went well. I enjoyed being back in London but very soon I realised how hard it was to make friends and be part of the London scene. I was living on my own, going shopping and swimming, but really had no other hobbies.

All my London friends had gone off elsewhere. I remember looking at our window- dresser and being so envious of her job. She seemed to dance in and out of the shop weekly, dressing the models, having a life with her boyfriend, and just being happy. Soon it took over me and I couldn't cope. I dissolved in floods of tears and had to ask my father to come back and help me return home.

Back in Loughton things were no different. I fell into deeper and deeper depression. I remember a dear friend from the old days coming to see me and how lovely it was. I was in such a state I couldn't even wash my hair.

During this time my parents had decided that with my father's retirement they would try to move to Suffolk. They helped my grandmother pack up her flat and found a light modern bungalow just out of town. This was perfect for my parents. When my Dad was in medical training, we had lived in Seattle for two years when I was 2. There they had seen many similar bungalows and loved them.

At least this was a change and a new beginning. I learnt how to drive at last and began to get to know a few different people from the area. I found life hard as I had lived such a colourful exciting life in Australia. Suddenly I was in a small fishing town, albeit with nice cafés and cinema.

There were many ex-Londoners who had brought business to the town which helped.

After a few months I found a flat in Leiston, close by.

I was ready to handle Life again, I thought.

⸺⸱◅◆▻⸱⸺

Chapter 7

Steve

One night I went to see a band on my own just to mix with some different people and hear some music. It was here I met Steve; he was playing lead guitar that night in his group called The Naff Band. Steve and his ex-wife had a daughter called Charlotte who was 8. He lived in East Bergholt Ipswich, in a commune, and worked in a day care mental health facility. We had a connection, but I don't think I was really seeing clearly.

I had recently had an upset at a job when I was working at a café in Aldeburgh. I got very high and had to be hospitalized for the night. My father had a doctor friend who advised him that I might do well to start taking Lithium, as I had had psychosis in Australia too. I think it was early days for this medication to be used, but over the years it has been a life changer for me.

In the beginning my weight might have fluctuated but I have been quite slim for a good number of years now. As I write, I have been taking it for 37 years. My advice to anyone is to take it consistently. You might feel recovered and in control wanting to stop, but nearly always the mania comes back and results in being sectioned or hospitalised. Usually after this, probable depression and loss of one's job could follow.

It is utterly awful.

When taking Lithium, you are monitored every 3 months to make sure your kidney, thyroid, and other organs are doing well (a simple blood test.) This is all you need to know that everything is on track.

It was worrying to me that I might lose my creativity and heightened feelings if I stayed taking lithium permanently. But I have found myself a much more stable person, enjoying a full life and much better personal relationships. I painted my T shirts well into my 40's and still enjoy painting as a hobby.

I regress….

I kept seeing Steve and looked for a nice house to buy in Ipswich. With my grandmothers help financially, I found one near the city centre. It was liberating.

Steve helped and supported me. He made me shelves and a kitchen bar. I had fun being a groupie to his band and made some great friends.

But there were problems….

I didn't realise that Steve was an alcoholic. So, with both of us not well, we had a very tumultuous relationship. I did love him at the time, but it was very difficult. He would come back from work, and I could tell if he'd been drinking. I would find empty cans of special brew in cupboards. We had terrible rows. One holiday we had together, we were on a flotilla in Turkey with my father and I got pregnant. I knew this wasn't the right relationship to be in to have a child and coupled with the fact that I had recently started on lithium, which could hurt a child's heart, I had an abortion. This was not difficult for me as I felt it was the right thing to do, but very sad.

Steve and I had two years together, we did get married, but it didn't help.

During the last months of our relationship, he got close to a lady in Ipswich, who was also a drinker. So we parted amicably.

Chapter 8

Ipswich

Business

Her speciality is Technicolor dream coats — with style

DESIGNER Cathie Nairne has just returned to Ipswich after running a successful business abroad hand-painting T-shirts and sweatshirts.

Strong individual patterns and bright colours are the hallmark of Kats Designs, which is now based permanently in the town.

Sweatshirts

Cathie, who originally comes from Ipswich, came up with the idea of hand-painted T-shirts and sweatshirts for children and adults while she was running a stall selling Indonesian clothes in Paros, Greece.

"First I tried tie-dying and painting characters on the shirts using the strange shapes from the process as background. Now I am picking out the most successful designs and painting them directly

onto T-shirts and sweatshirts," she says.

Cathie, who is assisted by boyfriend Johnny Davies, has already had success in selling the designs at a number of London markets, and now she plans to sell them to various retail outlets in Ipswich.

"A number of shops in Ipswich have already shown interest in the designs, and I am also taking individual orders for Christmas. If anyone has a particular idea they would like to see on a T-shirt then I am happy to do it," she offers.

Brightness

"I think the main appeal of the clothes is their brightness and the fact that no two shirts are the same. Also there are no problems with washing because all the colours are set."

Anyone interested in Kats Design can contact Cathie on (0473) 252502.

PRODUCTION LINE: Cathie Nairne creating more of her hand-painted T-shirts

East Anglian 1992

I stayed in the house in Ipswich. I had friends from Steve's band and friends who lived very near, so I felt well supported. I don't know if Mum and Dad really supported my relationship with Steve, but they just wanted me to be happy. I didn't see them a great deal at that time.

I remember getting ill just at the end of the relationship and having to go into hospital, just until the lithium kicked in. Maybe I had forgotten or tried to reduce my pills. I have learnt after many tries here and there to reduce the lithium, but it never seems to work. After say, a week, you start feeling high, your diet changes to wanting food and drink you wouldn't normally consume. I wanted to smoke, which I had virtually given up by then.

You feel very psychic at first, and alive, but if it continues you spiral out of control. It's then that you need help and the unfortunate outcome is the depression again.

I had various jobs in Ipswich. The longest being in a health food shop called Fruits of the Earth. I met a lovely friend called Caz, who I still see today. She supported me and was lovely to talk to.

We started driving down to Camden to sell her beautiful silver jewellery. I fell in love with Camden market. It had been a few years since I have been in the environment of a thriving, joyous, colourful market, and I loved it. All I wanted to do was find an excuse to work there myself, with something that I was producing. But we could only go at weekends if we were lucky enough to get a stall.

I had a habit of getting bored. I decided I would love to go to a Greek island and asked my close friend Mandy to join me on a trip to Paros in Greece. I had always loved the Greek islands. Holidays from Monsoon with Jo were nearly always there.

After a short flight, we took a ferry to the islands. The intense sun and cobalt blue sky just washed over me and everything seemed perfect. We stayed in a small cottage and spent our days on the beach or at a café making friends. When Mandy had to leave, I decided to stay on a short while longer. I found a dance studio that I fell in love with and asked the landlady to hold it for me, giving her a deposit, saying that I would finish my job and come back.

This I did, but when I returned, I found a Welsh man had barricaded himself in the house which was rather startling. With the help of some friends including a brilliant Spanish man (or rather actor), we managed to put the fear of God in him, and he left, leaving me to enjoy the cottage with friends who came to visit.

This was a marvellous time for me. I started painting on T-shirts. It all came about when I met a man returning to England and selling his paints and T-shirts. At first I didn't know what to paint on them at all. I found some peppers which I cut up and dipped into the paint, but soon I remembered the Easter Island heads I drew at school, and I also started painting what I saw around me.

Soon I was getting rather good. I sat on the pavement and painted, and passers-by would ask me about my work and occasionally buy something. The Greek shopkeepers didn't seem to mind me painting on the street too much, but soon I went and joined other traders in a market/ bar in the evenings.

I worked hard and loved it. In a few weeks my friend from Ipswich, Caz came over to spend a couple of weeks with me.

During this time, I had met a nice couple in a bar, and we had become friends. A few people we knew had been painting on stones and attaching them to leather to make necklaces and we decided to make them too. After a short while the girl decided she didn't like me and refused to talk. It was hard for her partner who couldn't understand what was going on. At the end of the season when they were about to leave Greece, she rushed towards me, arms outstretched and begged me to forgive her. I was dumbstruck. Was this because of something I'd said, or my bipolar? I never knew.

I tend now to give new friends a wide berth. To love them as much as possible but rely on myself first. I realise my behaviour can be different from others sometimes.

After a couple of months, the weather was getting cooler, and the tourists were going home. A Greek guy who had been making advances for a while, asked if we could become more than friends. I decided that it might be fun to hook up and eventually he came back to England with me.

I had a friend looking after the house, so everything was fine there. Dimitrious (Dimi) enjoyed England at first but soon got tired. He started painting madly in my cellar, but we didn't have much in common. I put on about two stone in weight, I think because we just couldn't communicate.

So, he left and went back to Paros.

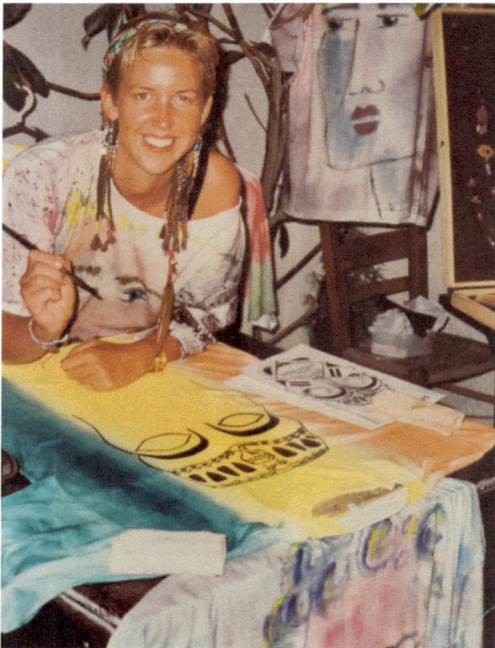

Paros, Greece

Chapter 9

Amsterdam

During this time living in Ipswich, I had various small jobs but was still restless and looking for more adventure. One day I packed up some clothes, took my bike and boarded a ferry at Harwich, sailing to Amsterdam. I went by myself as a friend was looking after my house, and I had a friend who was already over there. My aim was to stay with her, but in truth I only stayed with her a couple of days as it felt uncomfortable when her boyfriend arrived.

When I arrived in Amsterdam and had just left the train station, I met a boy called Laurie. We got talking and soon became friends and lovers. He introduced me to a friend of his who was running a rubber clothing shop in the red-light district and soon I was helping in the shop.

I felt quite uncomfortable wearing one of his rubber dresses. At the time it was an adventure I guess, and I had these new friends. Though they totally used me.

One evening I was the coat-check girl at one of his parties.

I marvelled at the folk coming in, dressed to the nines. Like the suited businessman who came out of the loos in a full gimp mask and rubber outfit.

I wasn't interested in all the S & M going on in the dance hall, but I did meet a wonderful transvestite. We talked for a long time. She was married and had children.

She had told her wife that he/she felt this way and her wife had accepted this. She invited me and her wife to a party made up of about 100 transvestites in the city. We must've been the only two women there. The group were mainly dressed very conservatively if I remember. Wearing twinset, pearls and wigs and looking very genteel.

I found myself being very wrapped up in Laurie. Living with him and helping him pack marijuana so he could put it on his body and take it back to England. Quite unbelievable to me now.

One night with a group of friends we took some ecstasy, and I totally went to another planet. I remember dancing madly to 'I've Got the Power' by Snap, on MTV. Lorie and I made silly dreams of buying a dog and taking it back to England and setting up Home. He was not the sort of person I would ever want to do that with in the real world. The night didn't end well, I remember being quite ill. I must've called my father because he tried to come over to find me, but to no avail. I did go back to Ipswich, but one day, at my friend Lisa's house, I tricked everybody (including my father who had come to help me). I ran away, with Lisa and family calling out for me to come back.

I got a taxi and a flight and returned to Amsterdam just using my credit card. Everything went wrong. Laurie had had enough, and I had to return home.

Lisa and I still laugh about it now!

This is the life of somebody who is bipolar and taking recreational drugs, maybe not taking their medication, and becoming out of control again. I was a really good liar, I felt I could do anything that I wanted and nobody was going to stop me. When you have a psychotic attack, you have very strange mixed-up thoughts and emotions and can damage yourself quite easily because you are so headstrong. I saw images and did some extraordinary things, which could have been fatal.

I also remember meeting an Egyptian man when I first arrived in Holland, who helped me find somewhere to live. My friend Jane and her boyfriend were not available, and I didn't have a lot of money. He helped me find some people who let me stay as a lodger.

I remember him helping me move an old TV inside and struggling to get it up the stairs. We saw each other as friends for a while and I was very grateful for his help.

I got a complete shock when I returned to Ipswich. He called to ask me whether I would marry him as he wanted to stay in Holland. He offered me £1,000. After some thought, and as I was short of money, I agreed and went back over to Amsterdam.

Completely crazy.

It took a while to set up, but I was very naïve. No one knew. We got married, but it was never consummated, we were just friends. The authorities soon picked up on this deception and I was called to see the police. It was all quite frightening. After a short talk they let me go. I was lucky, but he was deported.

Chapter 10

Camden

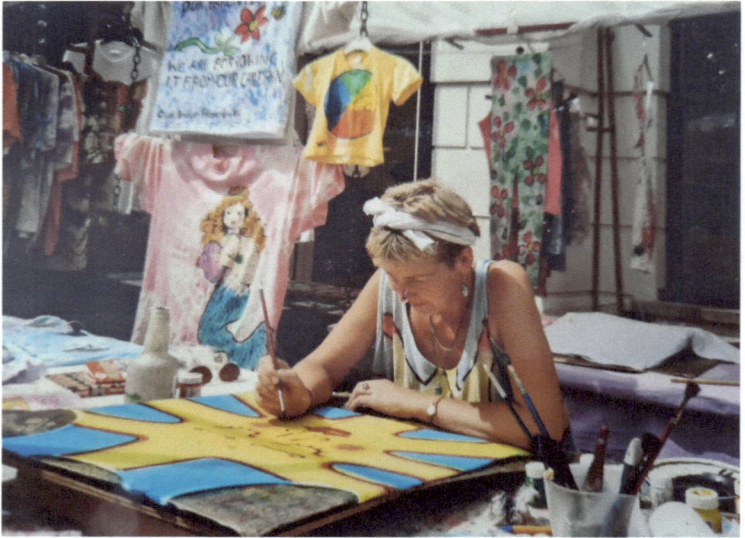

Camden

Back in Ipswich I went back on my medication and resumed a relatively normal life. I had loved the time In Camden in London and decided that if I stayed at my brother's house in Brick Lane, which was empty at the time, I would be able to work at the market. My parents were quite worried about my going out in London at night but, as I was in my 30s now, I felt perfectly safe. I had lived in Sydney for almost 3 years on and off and learned a lot about life and danger.

I started working inside at Camden market and loving it. I painted there whenever I could, on T-shirts mainly, although I did sell cards that I had made previously in Australia.

One day a boy came through the market. I saw him from a distance as I had been washing my brushes in the toilets. I just knew that we would connect. He was looking very earnestly at my work, and I found out later that he was a glass painter and had been accepted on the Princes Trust.

Tufty lived near Camden at the time, and we started seeing each other. He had many tattoos and was dressed in black. He had been in foster care growing up in Lancashire where he had had a rough time, but we could talk deeply, and it felt good. He was extremely artistic and a loner.

He made a platform bed in his flat so that we could sleep together and helped me a lot at Camden market, especially climbing high to advertise my T-shirts all over the rafters. I loved him at the time, but it was very difficult because he was so different from me and my parents found it awkward. We were together maybe two years but by the end it was getting too hard. He preferred marijuana to food at the time, I think. I just found it all very frustrating. Also, being around the smoke was affecting my health.

We planned a holiday in Australia. It was very difficult getting him a Visa because he had been in prison for a short time for stealing cars, but we got there. Silvia showed us around and we had a wonderful time. I remember him seeing a sign saying Welcome Home Johnny, (his original name), which he found very profound!

Back in London I had another psychotic episode and unfortunately, I had to be sectioned. I remember the policeman coming to take me to the Whittington Hospital in Archway.

It was very strange being there all alone. I saw poor people obviously struggling, rocking on their beds. I responded to my Lithium quickly and luckily met a lovely couple who were assisting the nurses, who befriended me.

I can't remember my parents ever coming to see me. I imagine my father was too busy. But Tufty and his friend Miles came once or twice. After about 3 weeks I was allowed to return home.

Eventually it all broke down. One day in a fit of anger, Tufty raised a T-square ruler over my head, which I ducked. I think it might've killed me.

That was the end, I decided to pack up my things. With my cat, Sheba, on top of the luggage, I drove down to Bristol to stay with Mandy.

Chapter 11

Bristol

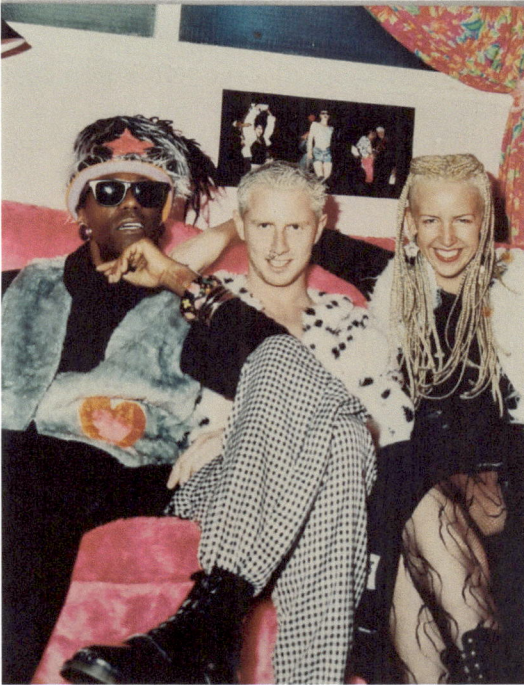

BS8 Bristol

I couldn't stay in Mandy 's flat very long. She was living with her boyfriend Andrew, and I felt in the way. Eventually I found a flat in Redland. I had my own space even though it was quite small. And they took pets. I did love living in Bristol especially at the beginning. It was colourful and alive and reminded me of being in Australia. Shame about the weather!

I was able to work in Saint Nicholas market painting my T-shirts.... I felt free and liberated.

One day I was painting and I noticed a very carefree, happy young man with short dreads in his hair and I asked him where he got them done. This was the beginning of a great friendship with my gay friend Nick. I hadn't had wild hair since Australia. In Sydney dreadlocks were very trendy especially with Boy George and a new look that he had created. That time I had dyed my hair black and had dreadlocks sewn in, with orange painted sides to my head. It was a strange look, but great fun. Nick said he could put in blonde extensions to my hair, and I loved it. I was suddenly introduced to his group of friends. I felt I belonged.

We styled each other's hair and went clubbing. I was introduced to Sapphire, who was a great light in the club scene. He lived on Gloucester Road and walked the streets in women's clothes with the attitude of a supermodel!

Later on I was to help run a shop inside a bunch of shops, called BS8, on Park Street. Paul, Sapphire and Nick all helped me set up the shop with Jules, who was previously my landlady. I did laugh when Paul suggested we call the shop Bitch!!

It was fun, every day we dressed up and enjoyed being there. Paul and I were painting and Sapph had fluffy waistcoats made for sale in the shop. As much as we loved it, we didn't sell much. I think we only lasted three months.

By now I had a house of my own in St Pauls. It was very near the famous Black and White café where there had been shootings a few years before. But I never felt afraid. When I left the house, with my funky hair and large DM boots, I felt invincible.

One day I met Tom. Probably in his late 20s whereas I was about 35. He lived in a small flat on Ashley Road, which was in complete chaos. But I felt at home with him. I loved his carefree and childlike presence as we skipped down the street. We ended up working together a bit, he was making clothes while I painted my T-shirts. Tom was very talented, unsophisticated, just a real raw talent.

When my uncle Andrew died, he left me some money and we decided to go to India. We arrived in Delhi and made our way up to Pushkar in Rajasthan. India was amazing, like being on a film set, but we didn't get on that well some of the time. We got terribly ill at one stage when we were on a train. I fell on the floor of the loo, which was only a hole in the steel floor of the train. I was concussed and tried to find my way back to Tom but fell again and hit my head badly. I remember Tom having to clean me up and a lovely Indian lady, sitting opposite us on the train, rubbing my head and soothing me with oils.

I needed a wheelchair to leave the train at a stop that we didn't recognise, and having to find somewhere to stay the night. I do remember feeling better and going into the bathroom but got a shock when I saw a hole in the wall and an eye looking back at me!

I think we had a few weeks there but were glad to get home.

Tom and I met some new friends through a healer we met at a festival. Bernie was a lovely man, and I liked his presence and what he taught us. I joined a group of friends, and we would go to small retreats he arranged.

We practiced different healing techniques on each other and experienced some guidance and peaceful spiritual discussions. There were many festivals around Bristol, and I loved camping. One time we took all my finished t-shirts to Wales to a big outdoor festival. It was a great atmosphere until the heavens opened and we got soaked!

During this time I had gone to London to see how Tufty was getting on. Unfortunately he looked terrible, and I decided to help him move to Bristol by exchanging his housing association flat. He was hardly eating, and I was quite worried. Eventually this worked and he settled in a nice flat and found a rescue cat. Unfortunately, he was not at all stable and one evening I was called to find him in hospital as he had attempted suicide. He really felt that he had no real friends, as I had left him to live back with Jules. Thankfully there were more people around who cared for him, and he slowly recovered. We have stayed in touch from time to time, on Facebook. It is lovely to feel he is ok and doing well.

I did have other boyfriends, but nothing really worked until Tom, who I saw for maybe two years. When we split up, I was very unhappy and decided to move to Glastonbury. Tom 's parents lived there, and we got on well. I found a house in Chilkwell Street which was perfect. It had three floors and felt enormous for just me.

I did have some connections in Glastonbury. During my time in Bristol, I had met a nice couple who had a stall at Glastonbury Festival. Luckily, they had an opening in their shop, Bedlam, and I was very lucky to accept a little job there. Also, it was great to meet people. Soon I met Chris, a psychiatric nurse and Jo, who also worked for the NHS. They married and have remained great friends through many ups and downs, even helping me through a delusional episode.

Glastonbury is a very special place, not just for alternative ideas and crystals. The energy here is powerful and the lay lines cross on the Tor, a must climb with stunning views.

I worked at Glastonbury festival for a few years on my friend's stall, on the Green-fields.

There is nothing like this wonderful festival. Seeing all the different events, installations and incredibly creative people absolutely blew me away. And, of course, the music.

Back in Chilkwell Street I felt uneasy. Sometimes I felt very lonely and could hardly answer the phone or answer the door. But this passed with the help of good friends.

I had all this space and wanted to share. Some friends introduced me to a lady who needed a room, and I decided to have a flatmate.

Unfortunately, she had an illness like mine and things didn't work out. She had a child that she had left with her ex-partner and found life very difficult with depression. But she did stay for a few months until things just got too much.

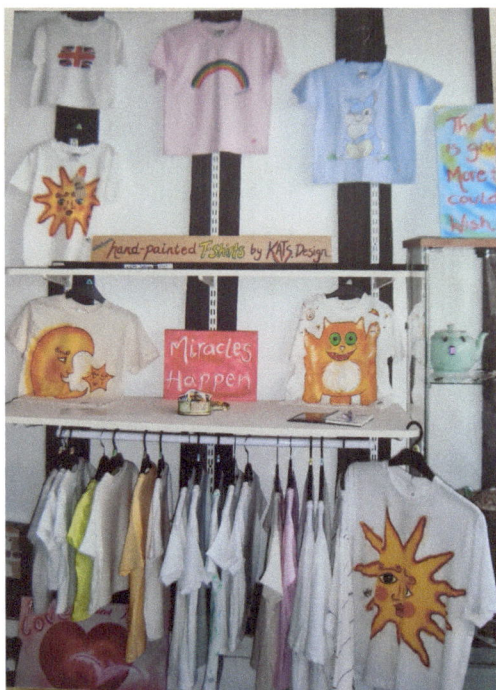

Waterfront, Ipswich

Chapter 12

Dion

A few weeks before I had met a wonderful stranger at a Halloween party in the Town Hall. Dion was exceptionally good looking. He was 6' 5, he had long flowing black hair and beautiful skin. I was 39. He was 21. I honestly thought I was much too old for him, but I was very attracted to him.

Later he came back to my house with a friend of mine, and a connection was made. Funnily enough I had dreamt of meeting somebody with long black hair.

When I lived in Bristol, I kept seeing men who looked like Anthony Kiedis, the lead singer of the Chilli Peppers, and other such personalities. I dreamt of meeting somebody like the men I'd seen at the festivals, creative and colourful with ribbons in their hair. So when I met Dion he just looked the part ... and the connection was strong.

Dion had had a bad trip on the Tor, and friends said that he wasn't very well. That he had become very inward, and his personality had changed. I don't remember seeing that side of him much. We just got to be good friends which turned into a relationship. I was older but it didn't change anything. He was affected by smoking joints, so I suggested he give up; that made all the difference. Also, they affected me too. He was a lovely person and kind.

He moved in quite quickly. He had been living with his family, not far away. They were humble and loving people who adored him but had been worried about his health.

Dion helped me ask my flatmate to leave. She threatened suicide but was soon coaxed out of her room and went to live down the road with a friend.

I loved that house. It was three storeys ... with a big bedroom for us at the top. I often took lodgers in before that encounter.

One afternoon I came home to find about six boys, all friends of my lodger, watching porn in the living room. I hastily asked them to leave!

Another day a lodger got a phone call from Australia and completely forgot he had left the bath running. When I suddenly saw water pouring out of my light fitting, I realised what was happening ...

I preferred life without lodgers!

Dion was at Strode college. He asked to photograph me in the nude, in agreeable positions, in our living room. I had long hair extensions at the time and the black and white photographs came out beautifully. But I did get quite a shock when I went to the open day at the college and saw my images in huge display all over the walls of the Art room!

It wasn't always easy. Although Dion had had a relationship with an older lady before, this was still challenging. But we supported each other, talked about everything and I helped him to drive. We loved working with our friends at Glastonbury festival, roller skating, and time out with family. But we did have heated arguments.

After about 3 months of being together I was looking for a holiday in Spain or Portugal. The lady on the phone just offered me a week in Las Vegas. Dion had never flown; it was all very exciting.

My friend Sarah said, "You'll get married!" and that put the idea in our heads .... It wasn't planned.... but we did get married in the Little White Chapel, a venue chosen by many American celebrities. The celebrant was so sincere, and it was a lovely service.

We had the best time; we were very happy together and were fascinated by the city. We took our roller skates and skated round the car park. We saw a show at New York, ... we ate burgers in the diners and went to the Hoover Dam. Sadly, we missed the Grand Canyon due to foggy weather....

On return our families got quite a shock. I think my parents were used to my impulsive behaviour but it was difficult for Dion's family. However, they were supportive as we were very happy together at the time.

We enjoyed living in Glastonbury, and after college finished in the summer, flew to Greece for a two-month holiday. Dion had decided to take up a media course at Bristol university. We decided to sell the house, and found another in Bedminster, South Bristol. It was a bit of a rush to find it and it was quite small but perfect as a start.

Towards the end of the course, we were travelling through Exmoor. Alone in the vast expanse of countryside I suddenly had a fantastic idea... "Shall we go travelling for a year ... to experience several countries...?" I asked. Dion wasn't sure at first, but it seemed to me to be the perfect time.

We bought Around the World tickets and packed a huge rucksack .... we planned to visit India, Nepal, Vietnam, Australia, New Zealand and Fiji, before ending in California.

We did it.

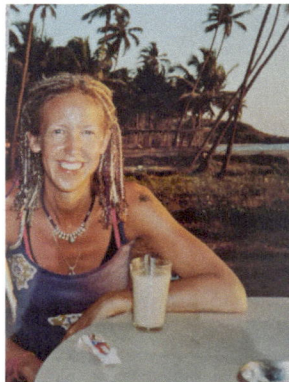

Nepal

Sometimes it wasn't easy but all in all we had an amazing time. We had various upsets but usually managed to talk it through and understand what was going on and fix it. We are both spiritual people who have made an effort to understand ourselves and get the most out of life. Problems usually started if I had missed my lithium. At one time, in Glastonbury, I remember trying to cut down my dosage. I got very upset and imagined strange things during my psychosis.

For example, believing Michael Jackson lived in the house opposite or having to destroy all my CDs as they were not the right music. I also became very upset when Dion tried to help me.

This incident resulted in me having to go to hospital and what was so incredible was that when I got there I suddenly was back to my completely normal self, talking eloquently, and the doctors found no reason to hospitalise me. It was very difficult for the friend of mine who took me there, who was trying to convince them that I had been really ill and talking Gobbledygook!

When we returned home after ten months travelling, Mum and Dad picked us up. I remember thinking they looked older. Which of course they were and probably been very worried.

We decided to look for work in Woodbridge, not far away, in Suffolk.

We found a lovely flat, with Mandy's help again.

Dion worked in a delicatessen, but eventually he needed to work in media, and we rented a flat in Brixton for 6 months.

It was exciting to be in the city again.

I found part time work in a lovely clothing and gift shop in Blackheath. When I started, I got on very well with the owners. Unfortunately, I was soon joined by a new lady manager who took an instant dislike to me. She made my life extremely difficult as I tried to be helpful and be a good assistant as well as I could. In the end we had a huge row. I lost my cool after being pushed down too many times. Whether she took a dislike to the fact that I had managed Monsoon branches I'm not sure.

Dion found a good job, though, and otherwise we enjoyed being in London.

While we were living in Brixton, I saw an advert to join a small group on a Past Life regression course in Spain. I had to borrow the money from my Dad, who couldn't understand why I should think it would be of interest to me.

I remember him saying he thought I'd had a dreadful life…. I was aghast. I replied I had had an amazing life, so many adventures.

I have been interested in past lives for a long while, but I kept my thoughts to myself. I have a very open mind and have done a lot of self-discoveries. In India reincarnation is generally accepted and I so wanted to understand it more.

When I arrived in Spain, I was met by the most charming, older man, who had been brought up with eight sisters. He told me he wondered why I hid my light under a bushel. I was probably rather shy about myself and my life.

I liked everything he said about reincarnation, and it was fun to meet others who felt the same way about spirituality. We did various activities to ascertain what we might have experienced in our past lives. This included a deep relaxation session and being brought to the end point of a previous life.

I saw myself in Egypt at the side of a vast lake, I had black dreadlocks.. I told my companion, who was with me during the session, that my husband had been very cruel and beaten me, and that I had taken poison as I wanted to die. This was a very clear experience, and I can see the lake now in my mind eye.

Unfortunately, I got ill during all this. I remember wanting to smoke and my diet changing and the next minute I was in some strange places with strange visions. I was having another psychosis.

I don't remember feeling very much, except a strange face peering down at me (the doctor I think?) and that was a bit frightening!

I had to leave and fly back to England. Dion wasn't very happy at having to pick me up, but I was in one piece and then returned to our flat. Various community helpers came in to check on my behaviour until I improved. Apparently if you are bipolar, having this experience of regression is not good for the mind and can cause this reaction.

I think this was the last time I experienced mania. I realised the key to a peaceful life is to stay on the medication. Every time I had an upset like this, it put me back so many weeks either in hospital or at home, with lack of confidence or depression.

After we had completed the six months in Brixton, we decided to rent in Greenwich. It was great fun being in the centre, with the gorgeous park and naval buildings around us. Greenwich also has a good market scene and had a different atmosphere to Brixton. Dion continued his job, and we spent six months here.

The next step was a move to Dorset so Dion could do his MA in Bournemouth. We rented a flat in Bovington, where I found a part time job nearby in Wareham. I felt quite isolated at times. After 6 months I rented a small flat in Aldeburgh so I could visit my parents and a few friends from Bristol came down and enjoyed the glorious countryside in Dorset. It was a strange time as Dion had his own university friends, but it was only a year.

After this another move. We found a house to buy in Manningtree, on the High Street. Dion could commute to work in London, and I found a job in a contemporary whole food shop with lovely staff. It took a while to make friends again but as it was such a small town, it didn't take long.

After roughly a year, on his return from a week's course, Dion told me he needed his freedom and for us to break up. It was awful but I understood. We had tried to separate a couple of years earlier and I realised our age difference was too big. There was still a lot of love between us. At first, I was practical but eventually the shock and anger surfaced.

Dion and I had exactly ten years together. It seemed like a sign. A past life relationship we thought. We both 'saw' pictures in our minds of past lifetimes we could have shared together. I thought we may have lived in India.

We wondered if we may have had problems that had to be resolved in this life. Anyway, it was difficult for me to let go, but I was rational at the end and Dion went to live in London.

We lived in 8 different houses together, including 4 rented flats.

···◄═❮○❯═►···

Chapter 13

Running away

Mum and Dad were on their way to Canada to see my brother and his family. I decided to join them. Life had been difficult for me without Dion. I wasn't sure in what direction to go.

My brother Stuart lives in Vancouver and has now lived there for 36 years. He met Lietta, his wife, when doing medical training in London. My Dad and grandfather were both very high in the profession. But it's a huge commitment and not one to be taken lightly. He decided it wasn't for him and started working with computers, a job he still does today. Lee and my brother both share a love of sport and music. They became a couple and now have four girls in their 20s, who are wonderful, independent and well-travelled young ladies.

On the plane I was seated next to a pretty girl a bit younger than myself, and we saw that we were both reading the same book "Eat Love Pray 'the number one best seller.

This book especially appeals to recently divorced or single women, I imagine. We got talking and didn't stop for maybe five or six hours!

Kristin was recently divorced. She had a young daughter, Lola, who was about two. We both found we had lots in common and as the conversation progressed, she suggested that I come to San Diego as she had rented a flat there. This was very exciting for me as I wanted to escape for a while. During my holiday with my brother, I did go and see her where she was staying with her parents. Later I took a plane to San Diego, where I stayed with her for about six weeks. Kristin was madly Internet dating! She introduced me to a few of her prospective men, but I wasn't ready. We enjoyed California and the sunshine.

It was just too early to think of new partners. When I got approached in a bar by a sweet guy, (who looked a bit like my first husband) I just froze. I couldn't even talk to him. But I was so happy just to be out and about with her and her friends.

Next, I went on to a hostel in Venice Beach and then to Santa Ana to meet close friends of the family. After this I flew to Australia and met my friend Silvia in Sydney, then up the Gold Coast to see Nick, who had moved there a few years before.

Since this trip I went on two retreats taken by Kristin and her great friend Jonathan George, and my now husband, Paul. They were in Bali and Costa Rica, just a fabulous and healing experience.

I had always dreamt of being on stage miming like a drag queen. In Bali I got the opportunity! One night we decided to go to a small but famous, gay club called Bali Joe. My friends were surprised when I told them I wanted to have a go, and they arranged it! A quiet man led me upstairs and did my make-up. I was petrified! I couldn't talk, even when Kristin came to give me encouragement.

I was given a huge wig and thankfully my simple black dress was just right. The whole experience was brilliant. I loosened up on stage, dancing to Simply the Best by Tina Turner. What a night, even the locals approved!

Back to the story.... On my return from California and Australia I had to sell the house in Manningtree, where I had lived with Dion on the last stretch of our time together. I felt I had no choice but to go back to live with Mum and Dad and to help them as they were now reaching 90.

Chapter 14

Aldeburgh, again

After a while I found a new home in Friston, a small village ten minutes away from Aldeburgh, and found work in various pubs, before I found a better option.

The Pelican was a large restaurant mainly serving fish and chips. As Aldeburgh is a seaside town and I liked the set-up, I thought it would be quite fun to be a waitress here for a while.

My manager Paul became a good friend, and I felt part of the town. The restaurant belonged to the owner of the fish and chip shop in town. Although I could see he was a very disturbed man I became quite fixated on him. His wife died of Motor Neurone disease and he was drinking heavily. It felt like I just wanted to make things better for him, as I could see him spiralling downwards.

Unfortunately he had history of being a philanderer, and little did I realise the next victim would be me. In his defence I really wanted the closeness and the sex. But I did not realise how this continual behaviour would shatter my emotions. We started living together after I uncovered one 'affair,' and he wanted me close, but I kept the cottage in Friston. I must have left him about six times during this period but crawled back when he said he needed me.

This relationship went on for almost 2 years. We went to Jamaica, San Lucia and sailed in Greece. Believe it or not he was much better behaved on holiday, but in Aldeburgh he was King Pin and for a very shy man, actually had good relations with the locals. He was very generous in the pub.

One day my friend rang me up. She had seen him with another lady entering a clothing store down the High Street. Immediately I rang him up, he was now at work in the chip shop and distracted. I asked him if he was seeing somebody else and he said yes. That was it, I had had enough.

He had met her six months ago and had been seeing her on and off all this time. He had even taken her to the golf club dinner and displayed her as his new woman. I was ready to call it quits.

Later, I got very angry, and he did seem full of remorse. It was a horrible time for a while, but I did have support from friends.

Before our separation we went to lunch with my parents. My Dad hardly said a word, he could see this man was very bad for me. I only hoped this had not influenced his oncoming Alzheimer's.

My Dad went into a care home when he was approximately 92. My mother was very strong and knew she was doing the right thing when he started to soil the bed. It was a very sad time.

I had walked his Collie with him every morning around the Warren, a heath opposite their bungalow, for the last two years. One day he actually fell flat on his face and I thought he had gone. Now we think it was a small stroke. Sadly, he died in a care home in Bury St Edmunds two years later.

My Dad never said he loved me, but I always felt it. Nor did he tell me I looked pretty or well dressed. I wonder if this is a Victorian way, but maybe the reason why I looked for love and reassurance from men.

Soon we realised we would have to sell the house and my mother and I took it upon ourselves to start packing up everything. Luckily, we had a nice housekeeper and her husband who helped us a great deal. We rang Sotheby's and other similar places to get prices on some of the wonderful old china and glass my Mum had collected.

It was a huge operation. I was working part-time at Aldeburgh cinema; it was a busy time.

My brother came over from Canada to help for a couple of weeks. At last Mum found a buyer and it was time for her to move.

She found a flat in a sheltered housing establishment in Bury Saint Edmunds. This was very nice for me to visit as it's a lovely town, and I enjoyed taking her to lunch and shopping. We also went to visit Dad once a week. I spent a couple of nights on the sofa bed while I was with her and things worked out very well.

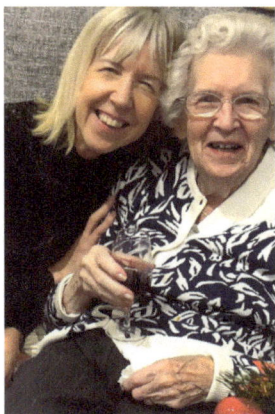

with Mum

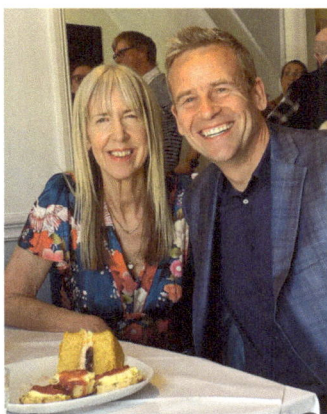

with Stuart

Chapter 15

Paul

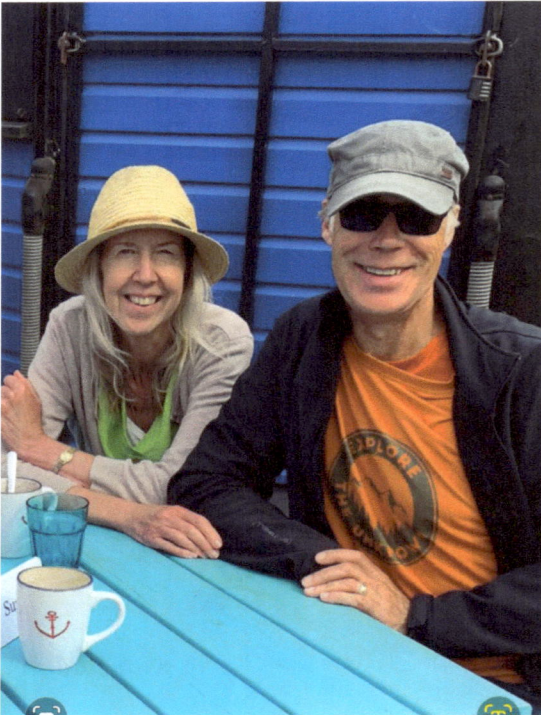

Cathie & Paul

One afternoon I was staying with Mum and looking through match.com. I had been working at Aldeburgh cinema for about five years and not met any prospective suitors. I did have a matchmaker at one stage. It cost £1,000.

I couldn't believe he didn't really come up with anybody suitable for that money! I met a range of different men all with something in common with me, for example India or Glastonbury Festival, but nothing gelled for me. One man even took me out to dinner and after the main course asked me outside for a breather. He then tried to kiss me there and then outside the restaurant. Just not my style!

My search went on for about 2 or 3 years.

Online dating is full of scams and false identities. I soon began to spot the scammers. Pigeon English and requests for money.

One afternoon I was with Mum in Bury. While I was looking on match.com, I saw somebody who reminded me of my cousin Mike. He wore glasses, which could've been why I suppose. We must've been looking at the same page on the phone because I connected with Paul very quickly and we ended up having a long conversation mainly about the awful time when his wife died.

We found it easy to talk to each other. He had had a terrible time dealing with circumstances around her passing. At the end of the conversation, I remember walking to my Mum 's bathroom and having the most extraordinary experience. I felt as if Wendy, Paul's wife, was talking to me, telling me she welcomed my presence and giving me the confidence that this was the right way to go.

We arranged a date and met up on Lowestoft beach. It was a glorious day but I remember getting lost to begin with, calling him and eventually finding the right place. I sat on a wall and watched his car drive down towards me. He was grinning from ear to ear. It felt a good start!

Paul was not what I expected. Being quite fashionable I was surprised to see he was wearing an old farming sweatshirt, old black jeans but quite nice black boots. His Norfolk accent was quite pronounced. But he was lovely.

He went very quiet for a while, and I tried to find out a bit more about his story. It was incredibly sad, about his wife contracting cancer and dying in their home. But honestly, I didn't think that he was the man I would marry, (though he did have a great sense of humour).

Paul worked on a farm near his home in Norfolk. He had also worked for a wood-working company, a horse charity called Redwings, and as a sous chef at a local hotel.

When we sat down for tea, it was hard to break through. We spent some more time together walking on the beach, and then went to find something to eat. Paul didn't pay for my dinner, which was fine but I was a bit disappointed. You never know how things are going to go, so this was the best course of action really. It wasn't till we got back, and I sat in his car to say goodbye that we both felt the urge to get closer, and then we couldn't stop!

We talked quite a bit on the phone and arranged to meet in a couple of weeks at my house in Friston.

The first thing we did was go upstairs! We got on very well (apart from not understanding his Norfolk accent occasionally!) Paul had the most terrible haircut too. Apparently, his brother had suggested it as he got so hot at work. But it didn't matter, he made me laugh and was very devoted. He came and met my Mum in the care home, and we went out to music nights at a pub nearby, where he met some friends of mine.

I had booked a holiday with a dear friend to Sardinia and had to say goodbye for a week. Shani and I had a marvellous time. It was a fabulous hotel, and we were able to glam up and feel gorgeous in the warm evening weather. When we came home, I had cold feet. I didn't know if Paul would want to dress up and go to the sort of events that I like to go to. His upbringing was very different from mine. So even though we had had such a fun time getting to know each other I decided to call it off.

My friend was very surprised as she had enjoyed meeting him at the music nights, and they got on well. I think I was just fearful of committing myself to another relationship after all I had been through.

Paul rang me on the phone very soon after getting my message and just made me laugh as usual. He would often repeat 'You'll never find anyone as good as me,' which I thought was very confident, so I swallowed my fear, and life began to go more smoothly.

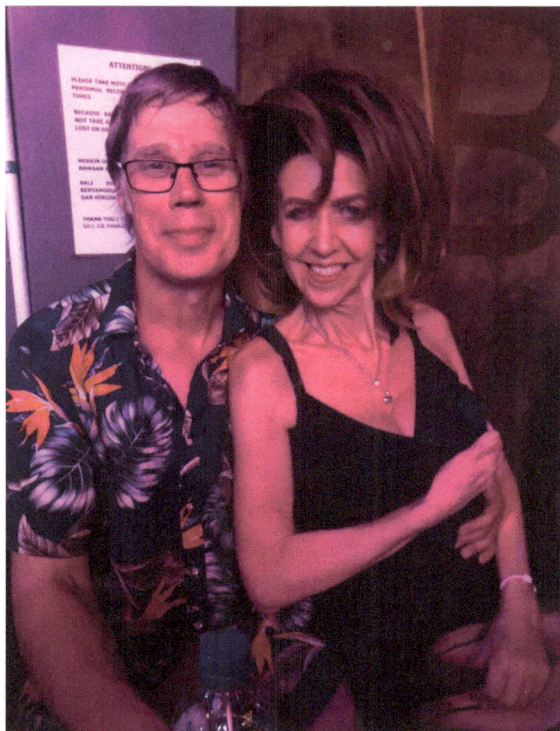

Bali

Chapter 16

Living together and tying the knot

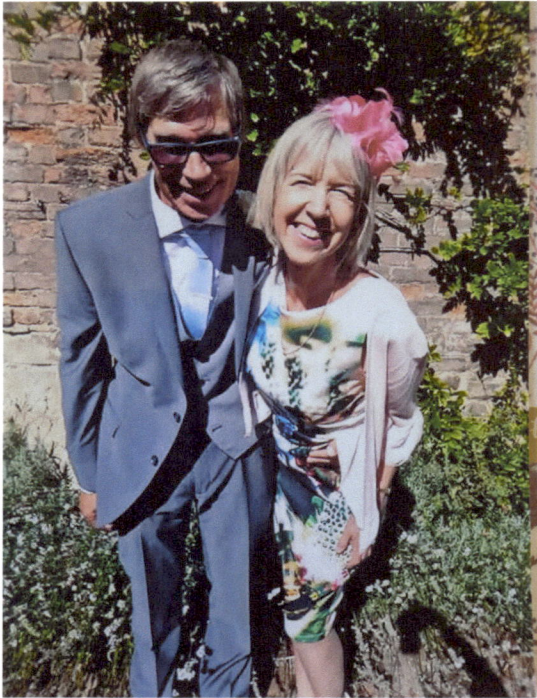

1st September 2017

I t wasn't long until I drove up to Norfolk to see Paul's house. He had a fantastic extension put on and I was very impressed with everything that he and his wife had been through to achieve that. Paul had taken on three jobs, and it was worth it.

The huge kitchen had a skylight and lovely conservatory, with a rockery wall outside and big garden. He had bought it as a small cottage, it was a terrific achievement. After his wife died, Paul waited about a year and a half before going online to meet somebody.

He told me that one day he sat at the kitchen table and thought, I need to share all this with someone, and that's when he went online. We both knew that life was better with a partner and things could be enjoyed more fully together. Also, I think with bipolar, although I was strong and capable, I had a very sensitive side and I found this world could be quite difficult. I wasn't always understood. I seem to be able to read people and see what's going on in a situation. Sometimes I feel impelled to try and make the situation better if I can, rather than ignore it.

Anyway, there I was in Paul's house. We had talked about living together and I had put my cottage on the market. There was no way I could move into the house as it was. Wendy had worked in a charity shop for the seals. She must've loved working there and many items had come back to the house. She was a very spiritual lady though and there were many interesting books like Nostradamus and Sai Baba. Being a similar type of person myself, I could identify similarities in our personalities. My favourite Guru, though, was Osho, whose ashram I had been to with Dion, in Pune India.

Also, there were photos of the two of them in the house and I had to ask Paul if I could remove them. We took a lot of the extra bits and pieces to the charity shops. I think we ended up with ten large bags.

All went according to plan, and I managed to get a buyer for my house, then I moved up to Norfolk.

It was fun getting to know each other better. The house was a field away from the cliff edge, with wonderful views of the sea. It was a special time. I dreamt of having a dog again. Every week I would drive to Bury to take Mum to see Dad and spend a couple of nights with her. She loved Paul from the start and was very supportive of our relationship.

I feel so very lucky to have met a man like Paul. He's very kind, sweet to my friends and loves animals. It shows you that what you wish for really does manifest. It just takes time. Never give up.

Our first house together was in Benhall, Suffolk. We found a perfect house for my Mum to join us. We enjoyed it immensely and I loved having Mum close. Paul found gardening work in Aldeburgh where my parents used to live.

Paul and I married in 2017... a joyous occasion, full of friends and family. We hope to be together for always.... with our two gorgeous dogs.

Marriage to me has been a real journey, believing there was someone who could love me forever.

I was blessed to find Paul. He is my rock and comfort every day. We have been married for 8 years on 1st September 2025.

We have already lived in 5 different houses, the first with Mum before she had to go to Bury St. Edmunds to sheltered housing. She moved again to Woodbridge after Dad died, and we followed her to be a support. Paul already had gardening work nearby. Then back to Aldeburgh, which was her final resting place.

We loved the Suffolk walks and to be near our friends again.

After she died, we decided to relocate to Somerset, first Wells then back to Glastonbury, where I had lived before.

Paul had never flown and had always wanted to travel. First, we travelled to Greece, then later to the Med on a cruise; Croatia and then the two retreats in Bali and Costa

Rica. I'm not sure we could handle an eighteen-hour flight again but never say never!

Recently we have discovered many new towns and cities in England. Loving Liverpool, York and Cardiff. With two dogs it is easier for us to drive, and we enjoy Cornish and West Bay beaches.

It really has been a great adventure. I have been blessed with the most wonderful friends, many of whom I still am in contact with. And we found our dogs, who mean the world to us.

I feel extremely lucky, I have my health back, and I have met Paul.

But most of all, I have found out who I am. I do have ups and downs, like anyone, but I now seem to make more logical decisions and feel so much calmer inside.

Music and dance have played a huge part in my life. I have lived through Rock, Soul, Disco, Ska, Punk, Hip Hop, Country and enjoyed classical music too, inspired by my parents, who loved Opera.

I have read that the happiness of one's life depends on the quality of one's thoughts.

I try and watch my thoughts and find more love in life every day. Accepting what I can't change but believing anything is possible.

I trust in the goodness of people and believe the universe is in our hearts.

I take Lithium every night and I haven't had a psychotic episode or mania for 20 years.

I feel I have mentally healed, as much as possible, and am clear and happy inside.

Loving Myself has been the key.

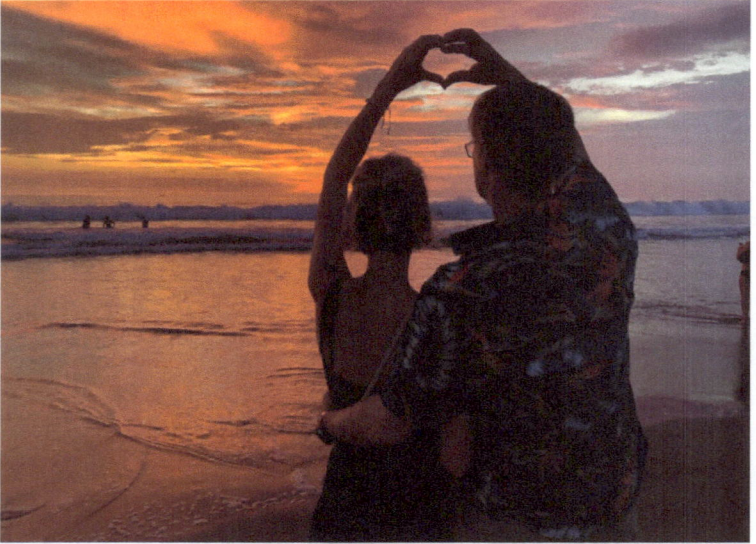

Costa Rica Sunset

So many thanks to everyone who has loved and supported me.

Books that inspired me:

Out on a limb by Shirley MacLaine

Jonathan Livingston Seagull, Illusions and Bridge Across Forever by Richard Bach.

The Prophet by Kahlil Gibran

Past lives and Future healing by Sylvia Brown (Includes past-life regression)

The Alchemist by Paulo Coelho

www.ingramcontent.com/pod-product-compliance
Lightning Source LLC
Chambersburg PA
CBHW041308020426
42333CB00001B/12